Antioxidants: How to Not Get Sick

I0439450

Table of Contents

How Our Body Relates To the War On Terror, A Cool Analogy

The world is starting to realize trends happen across the board. We're seeing trends in relation to political, social, and economic changes. This book is going to focus on changes that affect our health and wellness. Actually, we're going to only focus on one thing, antioxidants. Let's start with an analogy and an example to gain a slight understanding of how two opposing forces can affect our health.

Unless you've been hiding under a rock, you've surely heard about insurgents and radical groups taking over towns and villages. Some are even attempting to take over entire countries. Some of these radical groups will gain a stronghold of an area and slowly, but progressively move on to attack other areas.

The insurgents and radicals could have been in what we know to be "sleeper cells" and have been in that country for years. They also possibly invaded an area and come from a foreign country through borders that are less than adequately protected. As we saw in April of 2013 in Boston, Massachusetts they also could have been homegrown and warped mentally into being radicalized.

These groups can also do something equally as dangerous and frightening, they can encourage. They encourage others to follow their beliefs and activities and begin to grow, then, at rapid numbers and become far more difficult to defeat.

Is all hope lost? Not even close, depending on what sort of forces you have helping your country out! This is where a well trained and healthy army comes in, able to go right after the radicals and take them out, while carefully preserve and protect the honest and good citizens. Occasionally though, a country's natural defense is simply not equipped or has been depleted too greatly to defend against an ongoing attack. Is all hope lost? No, the country can call in mercenaries or other countries to help.

Do you see how this could possibly relate to your own body? Sometimes, especially in the case of my gorgeous niece who was born with Cystic Fibrosis, we are born with the insurgents already having a strong hold over parts of our body.

We could also have our natural defenses weaken by constant bouts of stress. Maybe we have a poor diet or are in an area where viruses and bacteria travel at great levels. Regardless, in today's age if the media is not talking about terrorism it is talking about the next epidemic or deadly flu strain.

I will not be overtly political in this short read, in fact I won't be political at all. I will however, go into some detail about why you need to know about the radicals that have a sole living purpose which is to infect you and make you ill.

More importantly, I will give you 20 known healing and preventing antioxidants to be anti-sick. These 20 antioxidants could help you fight infection and disease; they could help your body heal.

Relating to our short story above, these can help fight off the radicals, and help the local government regain control of their area! More importantly, these "special forces" have specialists that can also aid in DNA repair as well!

Free Radical Danger!

Going back to the story in the beginning of the book, I mentioned that there were radicals that can attack you (if you were a country). That is very true with your body, there are two main issues that can deeply affect your health and well being and truly wage war against your body and its systems.

There are more that can attack you and cause hell inside of you. Some are self inflicted (a lack of sleep, obesity, lifestyle related diabetes, etc.), and others are more environmental (think of things like fungal and bacterial infections). I'm focusing on one general and very dangerous, and not always preventable "enemies" or radicals.

The enemies you really need to concern yourself with are oxidative stress as well as free radicals, and they are extremely dangerous. Aside from being extremely dangerous, they can hit us on many different levels, at many different times, and they are not always noticeable until you find yourself in a severe world of pain! I'll spend a bit of time going over each one prior to finding out what we are using the 20 super antioxidants to fight against.

Free radicals are also known as oxidants which happen inside of or against aerobic (oxygen containing) cells. These cells create a natural balance through enzyme and non enzyme resources at their disposal known as antioxidants. Antioxidants are responsible for removing the threats of the oxidants. With that being said, it's crucial to have a balance of these guys in your cells.

It's not always, and doesn't normally, happen though - a perfect balance. When you have an imbalance some really nasty stuff can happen over time and it stems from something known as oxidative stress.

What kind of nasty stuff can happen due to oxidative stress? This is what helps cause aging, neurodegeneration (think Alzheimer's, dementia, etc.), cancer, and cardiovascular disease among other things. What causes this is mutations, damage, or changes to the cell molecules.

This could possibly confuse you, so I'll explain it more ineptly. Our cells (our own cells) produce free radicals. There's also some scientific acknowledgment to the fact that in some cases they can actually be beneficial to us!

A way to look at free radicals is to see them not as alien or bad intruders bombing us (although some of them can by nature). They should be seen in our analogy as regular citizens, normal everyday folks. But when they become energized, they cause problems. Energized states are what is thought to create the problem free radicals can deliver.

Who are known to cause problems on a regular basis? Let's look at a list of the reactive species that can cause harm in us:

- Singlet oxygen molecules
- Superoxide
- Hydroxyl Radical
- Hydrogen Peroxide
- Peroxyl Radical
- Organic Hydroperoxide

So what do these nasty sounding radicals attack? They can cause severe damage to proteins, DNA, and fats (lipids). These attacks can lead to some really (really) bad things such as carcinogenesis, mutagenesis, your enzymes could cease to function properly, and you could feel the effects of lipid peroxidation. Trust me; they're all really nasty and potentially fatal overtime.

Introducing Antioxidants: Why They Are Extremely Important To You

Antioxidants are naturally occurring compounds that fight off the harmful free radicals that can cause dangerous, and if untreated fatal, situations in your body. You can say, and be correct, that antioxidants sole purpose is to serve you. The way they serve you is by going out and killing off free radicals in turn helping to prevent disease.

Seeing free radicals can increase the aging process, it's often thought that antioxidants can help potentially reverse effects of aging, but at a minimum slow its progression.

Going back to the story at the beginning, these antioxidants come in different shapes, sizes, structures, and cover a very wide variety of roles. Think of them as an acting Special Forces group. When your body's natural defenses aren't enough, you may want to supplement with antioxidants.

So what do antioxidants do? The same thing as our special forces do (the analogy we're using), they neutralize and remove the threat posed by radicals. Some antioxidants don't just protect from and attack these nasty radicals, they also can aid in repair the free radicals may have inflicted!

Most antioxidants are thought to be free radical scavengers and come from a wide variety of sources consisting of herbs, enzymes, vitamins, phytonutrients, a particular hormone, and even a mineral.

Many antioxidants can be found in a healthy diet, but occasionally getting optimal levels strictly through diet can be near impossible. A reason for this is the soil that plants in particular come from. The soil is not going to be the same all over the place, in fact the nutritional value of the soil in my yard is different than that in my grandmother's, less than 20 miles away.

Alpha-Lipoic Acid

This antioxidant is pretty interesting in the roles it serves, and what's even cooler is the extreme benefit it can have on your health! This antioxidant is powerful, to say the least, has a VIP card of sorts (in regards to how it works in your body), it helps to "recycle", and it also stimulates other important things. Without giving too much away in the opening paragraph, let's look at how this "little guy" takes care of you.

Alpha-Lipoic Acid (we'll call it ALA from here forward) is extremely potent on its own. Let's touch on how it recycles after we gain an understanding on how we digest and use things we ingest. We take in vitamins and minerals daily, some need to be taken with fat and others are fine alone. These are fat and water soluble nutrients.

Certain cells require fats to work properly; this is where you need maybe some olive oil when consuming foods to allow the fat soluble nutrient to be absorbed. ALA is very flexible with how you can absorb it as it is both fat and water soluble!

Back to digestion, when your body is finished with a nutrient, it gets rid of the waste. Without getting into too much detail, if you go to the bathroom regularly you are witnessing first hand your body's "dumping" cycles of waste (for a lack of words).

There's a problem when we're dumping, and this is seen by trash pickers regularly. Sometimes we throw things out when we are not quite finished, right? This is where one of the roles of ALA comes into play with vitamins C (water soluble) and E (fat soluble). If there's still some use for them, your body prevents them from getting wasted so you can use more of these two vitamin forms of antioxidants. Think of

ALA as maybe more of a resuscitator than a recycler.

Probably one of the most important things that ALA stimulates internally is something called glutathione (read about it inside of Phytonutrient Superfoods and I bet you'll agree it's a pretty important antioxidant/amino Acid), and it also helps your body to absorb Coenzyme Q10. Both of these funny named things are extremely important to your body.

ALA may be new to you; however it has actually been used as a healing treatment in Europe for over 3 decades! In Europe it is used to aid in the treatment something really nasty called peripheral nerve degeneration. That's not all it does, and I have a surprise for you!

I mentioned that ALA has a VIP pass, recycles, and also stimulates, but it does something else as well that you should really appreciate. ALA also helps your body detoxify heavy metals from a very important part of your body. ALA can help your liver get rid of metal pollutants!

Are you really into ALA yet? You should be, and I'm not even finished talking about its helpful powers! It can help your body by protecting against the damage caused by oxidative stress on your nerve tissue. If cataract is something you fear or are already suffering from, ALA may aid in your treatments as well as potentially block cataract formation from even beginning!

Something I found very interesting came from a write up by Lester Packer a short time ago (yeah I'm a geek). In this, Prof. Packer (who also happens to be one of the leading antioxidant researchers) says he feels that ALA can also help us in fighting against some of the worst chronic degenerative diseases. He believes that supplementation may help fight and prevent things such as diabetes or cardiovascular disease (two major pains in the butt, well other areas but you get what I'm saying).

Speaking briefly of diabetes, ALA has already been providing some really neat benefits over in Europe. In parts of Europe, ALA has been used for some time now to aid in the treatment of diabetes. Specifically they use ALA to help control stubborn blood sugar levels in those with diabetes and backtracking a bit, some feel ALA treatment can help those with a prediabetic condition completely ward the condition off!

I mentioned that ALA is useful, if you're not completely sold into discussing it with your doctor here's a great reason. You actually may need it. I say this because without adequate levels of ALA in your system your body is not able to properly use sugar to produce energy. This leads me to wonder how large the correlation between a reduction in diabetic symptoms and supplementation with ALA really could be!

Our body can make ALA, just not sufficient amounts of it. You can get it through your diet by consuming things like potatoes, brewer's yeast, organ meats, broccoli, and spinach but even those levels are low. With that being said, taking ALA supplementally may not be a horrible idea. If there's any supplement in addition to what you're doing, I'd consider running this one by your doctor.

Bilberry

Have you ever been told to eat fruit instead of, let's say, ice cream or brownies? There's a good reason for that, ice cream and sugary foods common in American deserts (and unfortunately too common lunch boxes) make you fat (if you want to prevent that, check out Why You're Still Fat). Eating fruit and this should go without saying, is good for you and provides a ton of nutrients. In fact, blueberries are chock full of super powered nutrients!

Like blueberries, another potent herb/fruit is their European cousin, the bilberry. Europeans swear by the benefits of bilberry and apparently there's a lot of proof going into what they say! I first heard of this seemingly magical fruit while working for the nutritional company I mentioned. We were told it was one of the best supplements we had for a specific, and very regular, type of customer - diabetics.

We weren't specifically told why this fruit (many call it an herb) was so beneficial for diabetics and I am one of those people who need to know why. When I started researching it I was floored and amazed at what I read. Here's what I've learned.

I learned that diabetics are prone to some typical problems that can affect them on a multitude of areas. I found that diabetics can tend to have higher blood pressure, have unstable blood sugar levels, and are more at risk for venous or heart problems. Diabetics are also susceptible to getting nerve issues as well as healing problems due to an inability to clot. I'm glad I'm not diabetic!

Before I move on, there's a compound inside of bilberry called glucoquinine that has shown to aid in lowering blood sugar levels.

What this means is that the effects of high or low blood sugar could be greatly hampered!

Bilberry is amazing at helping things in our blood, specifically it aids us in two regards to our capillaries (and capillary walls). What it does is it helps the walls of the capillary become more fortified, meaning it makes them more flexible and strengthens them. It also aids in helping the capillaries more permeable for red blood cells.

What this does is it acts like a car going onto the freeway. If there's a blockage in the freeway, you're obviously going to have a far greater time getting into it, right? A compound in bilberry helps your red blood cells (cars) avoid those roadblocks and get right into your capillaries (highways). This makes the transportation of nutrients far more effective.

Like most other plants, bilberry has special compounds in it. These compounds are called phytonutrients (You really owe it to yourself to read about them here **Phytonutrient Superfoods**) do amazing things in our bodies.

One specific phytonutrient contained in bilberry are anthocyanidins, which are thought to have immense antioxidant properties in them. The reason this is something you want to know is what it can do for you. This phytonutrient, anthocyanidin, can help your cardiovascular system by lowering your blood pressure. It can also help your nervous system by aiding in enhancing the blood supply to it. On top of this, anthocyanidins can also help in clotting issues.

With its antioxidant properties, bilberry also has a lot of positive "anti" properties that are very beneficial to your health (and potentially even your appearance)! Bilberry can act as a pretty potent anti-inflammatory agent Inflammation is a damaging effect from free radicals, just like these two other properties we are going to look at quickly.

Aside from being anti inflammatory, bilberry and its compounds are also thought to possess anticarcinogenic as well as anti aging properties. What this means is that bilberry can potentially help your body fight off cancer cells from mutating healthy cells and drastically slow down the aging process.

We're almost finished with bilberry's benefits. I'd also like to mentioned that the phytonutrient, anthocyanidin, inside of bilberry is thought to be antioxidant in nature. How potent is it you may be wondering? Some studies (not one or two, but a solid handful) suggest anthocyanidins can be upwards of 50 times more potent than vitamin E and 10 times more potent than vitamin C.

Bilberry is something I helped make popular in the stores I covered, and although I was a sales associate the facts above gave me a conviction. If something is 50 times more powerful than a known antioxidant powerhouse, wouldn't you supplement with it? Something else you want to speak to your doctor about!

Burdock

You may just want to glance over this nutrient because it appears, and you're right, that there's a little information on it and that could take away from its power. Think about nature really fast, would you go and pick up a black widow spider because it looks small and harmless? Of course not, you know you'd die. Even though it's small in size it is extremely potent. The same goes for burdock.

This herb was looked into as, like bilberry, specific cultures raved about its healing properties. In fact, burdock is an oxide sniffing and killing machine! We know that superoxide and hydrogen peroxide are dangerous to us in the long-term, and now you will know that burdock has properties that can go out and scavenge for them.

Cancer that spreads is able to spread because of cell mutation, right? Burdock is thought (and believed) to help fight against that cellular mutation by controlling it. This could be a key reason why many cellular nutritional supplements (Flora, Daniel Chapter One's '7 Herb Formula' [which has helped me INCREDIBLY], and other top selling and popular supplements) contain burdock.

Coenzyme Q10

One of the first things that crossed my mind when I first heard of Coenzyme Q10 (we'll call it CoQ10) is that if nutrients had a secret agent, it would be this one! I also was prompted to look into what made CoQ10 so special in regards to cholesterol.

One of the first things I noticed when reading up about CoQ10 was that it came highly mentioned as being very beneficial for athletes. I had to know why as I was very active myself and found something interesting. I learned that CoQ10 was very important; actually that's an understatement in its role of energy production.

Your mitochondria are really small things in your body, but we already know that small things can pack massive punches and that is the case with mitochondria as well. Your mitochondria are your cell's energy production factories. How CoQ10 aids these little factories is by allowing them to use and metabolize fats and carbohydrates into sources of energy, or fuel. It also aids your cells in another area, it allows for your cell membranes to stay flexible.

That obviously didn't help me understand how it helped with cholesterol and aside from knowing it aided with cholesterol I was confused. Then I started reading more into various cholesterol lowering and managing medications and something smacked me (with knowledge, not physically). I learned that statins could dramatically reduce energy levels, and that started to make a ton of sense to me. CoQ10 helped promote energy production on a cellular level in your body which would counteract the effects of lower energy due to cholesterol lowering drugs.

That's not all I found out about CoQ10, in fact we know that cholesterol affects the heart, and that's the next bit of information relating to CoQ10's power I'll throw at you. CoQ10 is very beneficial for your cardiovascular system. In fact, CoQ10 concentrations are greatest in your heart muscle! I also found that in Japan, CoQ10 has been approved for treating cases of congestive heart failure (something that will kill you if left untreated).

CoQ10 has been known to act very powerfully as an antioxidant, but how exactly is where science appears to be slightly confused. One thing we do know (thanks to studies from South Africa and various places in Europe, and this is where it can be interesting) is how they believe CoQ10 can aid in the treatment of some severe health issues such as AIDS, cancers, allergies, and even muscular dystrophy.

Turmeric

Like bilberry, turmeric has a phytonutrient that provides some awesome health benefits. Turmeric is by nature, a spice and the phytonutrient it has in it is known as curcumin. Curcumin has a really special role, what this phytonutrient does is to prevent the formation of those nasty free radicals. It also aids in neutralizing free radicals that are already there. If you think about it and bring back our terrorism analogy, this antioxidant actually provides a primary and secondary line of defense.

I'll throw this out there because I want to get into why I am so interested in curcumin (and it is something I will not go without). Curcumin can stop the oxidation of cholesterol. What this does is it protects against the accumulation of plaque in your arteries.

This part is something that amazed me with curcumin and unlike most studies that have difficulties agreeing, they agreed across the board with this finding. I read into how curcumin acts towards cancer. Being a hypochondriac, I found this to be extremely interesting as I'm a heavy and very habitual smoker. Curcumin is believed to be able to stop precancerous changes to your DNA.

Do you remember that free radicals can inflame and eventually mutate our cells? There's a common knowledge that cancer is nothing more than, extremely dangerous, mutated cells. Right there we just learned that curcumin can stop them before they start causing all kinds of DNA changing havoc!

Staying on the topic of cancer, I'll also inform you that curcumin can interfere with the enzymes necessary for cancer to spread. While this isn't telling us that curcumin could potentially kill cancer, it is telling us that it could slow the cancer's progression.

Here's something that really got my interest, do you remember where I mentioned I'm a heavy smoker? If you're anything like me your mouth could hit the floor when you read this! There was a study into our kind, heavy smokers.

The study found that smokers who took a curcumin supplement (because it's difficult to find it in a grocery store) secreted less of something known as mutagens. If they sound scary, it is. Mutagens are substances that help cells to mutate. This was found by analyzing a variety smoker's urine. Either way we as smokers really need to quit.

Something interesting, but it's hard to beat that (said with a bias) is that harmful toxic compounds are seemingly blocked from coming near or bullying (touching) body tissue. I take this as also being able to protect against free radical damage.

Something curcumin does do, and if you're on medication that is anticoagulant in nature, is act as a blood thinner by stimulating bile secretion. If you take anticoagulants you're probably going to want to stay away from this nutrient unless your doctor strongly encourages you to take it. In that case, they'll probably be able to give you a safe level to focus on.

Flavonoids

I actually wrote a book on flavonoids (actually flavonoids and carotenoids) recently and you can grab it and read about them in Phytonutrient Superfoods. I'll be nice and cover how flavonoids can help you out here as well though.

Two things can be said and you'll find no scientific disagreement (if someday you do tell me as I am amazed when various scientists can agree with one another long-term) is that flavonoids are extremely powerful and potent metal chelators as well as antioxidants.

We mentioned defense, flavonoids actually act as the primary defensive mechanism for plants. They help the plants defend against bacteria, virus, fungus, This is normally a plant's only lie of defense and without it, the plant would obviously die.

Now knowing how this aids the plant, I will tell you it helps us in very similar fashions. We get our vitamins from plants, agreed? Flavonoids also aide the plant in protecting the vitamins from oxidative damage.

So what types of phytonutrients are out there? There are over 4,000 of them. But they d help in producing a variety of compounds, one of which we have mentioned (anthocyanidins).

Garlic

There are a few things I knew a little about when it came to garlic. One, my daughter and oldest son have loved saying "gaaaahlic" for years. I've also known it supposedly keeps vampires away. On a side note, when we went camping as youths we ate garlic ills as it was thought to keep mosquitoes, "chiggers", and ticks away. One thing I didn't know was how garlic acted in our bodies.

I began to understand it acts very well for the circulatory system. I had heard it can help to purify blood and that was about it. When I began reading how garlic, and a special form, of garlic could actually help as an antioxidant I was immediately interested due to my geek tendencies. I saw, as I really looked into it, some extremely impressive properties being discussed. What got to me even more was how the properties were being deemed as accurate in a variety of sources.

One of the first things I read wasn't what I had expected. I saw the first beneficial property of garlic being discussed in most sources in how it acts as a chelator. They chelate numerous heavy, and very toxic, metals so that the body is more able to excrete them. The particular compounds that handle this are known as sulfhydryls, which are a combination of sulfur and hydrogen.

Garlic also has the ability to help detoxify a variety of peroxides, such as hydrogen peroxide. Sticking with oxides for a moment, garlic has yet another oxide based ability. It helps in preventing fat from being oxidized which in turn helps in keeping the fat out of your tissues and arteries. That last tidbit showed a bit of the commonly known benefits of to the circulatory system.

Before I speak on a specific form of garlic, I will mention that garlic contains other antioxidant compounds in it. It has vitamin A, vitamin C, and selenium naturally. Each of these are potent antioxidants.

I mentioned in the previous paragraph about a specific form of garlic, the form is called aged garlic extract which I'll refer to as AGE through the rest of its write up. has had a whole bunch of various studies looking into its benefits, properties, as well as why and how it is like normal garlic on steroids.

The reason science is finding that AGE is so beneficial can be linked to the fact that it is the aging process that appears to refine natural garlic's antioxidant abilities. For instance, AGE compared to natural or "non-matured" garlic for example s its impact on DNA. AGE helps protect DNA from damage due to free radical "attacks"

As a plant, the phytonutrients (as mentioned in the write up on flavonoid) help protect the plant from environmental detriments. Plants need sun, however in life too much of one thing is not a good thing. That protection benefit also reaches over to humans when we consume garlic. Garlic is known to fight against radiation as well as sunlight damage. Interestingly enough, I did not see much in the way of being beneficial against skin cancer.

In general, the aging process of garlic in turning it into AGE appears to provide a greater concentration of the natural benefits of garlic.

Like natural garlic, AGE also aids in circulatory and heart health areas. AGE can help to reduce blood cholesterol. Additionally this aged form of garlic can prevent blood clots which in turn aids in protecting against and could lower your chances of suffering against heart attacks. Another way AGE can help ward off heart disease and especially heart attacks is by lowering the previously mentioned cholesterol levels in your blood. On the same note of elevated heart issues, AGE is also thought to be a contributing factor of maintaining low blood pressure levels.

One common drawback to consuming garlic is that it is the bad breath thought to keep away vampires. Although garli does have that effect, supplementally there are numerous products that have what is called enteric coating (popular with fish oil supplements) that help prevent a smell and aftertaste. There are not however, many medical (adverse reactions to medicine) attributed to a diet rich in garlic.

Ginkgo Biloba

Ginkgo Biloba is an interesting antioxidant and plays a great role outside of helping prevent you from getting sick. It's antioxidant properties are known to help individuals fight off free radical attacks, however in certain parts of your body. That is what makes ginkgo interesting as most other antioxidants are more free ranging than being focused on specific bodily areas.

Ginkgo, however, is known best not for its antioxidant roles but rather its brain enhancing benefits. When it comes to memory problems, even a novice in herbal medicine will probably mention ginkgo biloba as being a first choice in helping to enhance memory.

Although ginkgo biloba is greatly known for its memory boosting abilities, there's an area where we could see ginkgo being more accepted in mainstream media. Studies have been showing more and more that a massive strength in ginkgo is how it can have a positive effect in stroke recovery, lessening the effects of dementia, and also having a positive impact in the slowing of Alzheimer's progression.

Ginkgo has been known to aid in the circulatory system by enhancing blood circulation and the heart's effectiveness at pumping the blood. Speaking on ginkgo's ability to circulate blood, this also makes ginkgo potentially dangerous to individuals who take a blood thinner or painkiller by prescription.

Glutathione

Glutathione is another interesting antioxidant. It's not an enzyme, an herb, or even an amino acid but rather a protein which is created by 3 other amino acids. Glutathione is known to be extremely effective in protecting your body against free radicals damaging your cells.

In addition to protecting your cells from free radical damage, glutathione has also shown an ability to prevent the formation of free radicals from taking a stronghold in you.

As a smoker, glutathione could potentially be a life saver as it protects against the damage caused by cigarette smoke. In addition to protecting smokers, those who face exposure to radiation can also receive cellular protection through glutathione. Similar to radiation protection, glutathione has also been shown to protect against the havoc caused by chemotherapy in your body.

If you're wondering how glutathione protects your cells (which is a major issue in radiation and chemotherapy), the answer is a bit complex. In fact, unlike many nutritional supplements glutathione protects cells in a variety of ways. Take for example oxygen molecules, glutathione neutralizes them before they can damage or harm your cells.

Aside from protecting your cells through neutralizing them, glutathione is also known to work in conjunction with other antioxidants such as selenium. When paired together with selenium, glutathione has the ability to transform into a totally different compound. When selenium and glutathione combine they form something called glutathione peroxidase. This compound then goes after hydrogen peroxide and defeats it before it can cause cellular damage.

Aside from killing off free radicals and protecting cells on its own, in addition to transforming into a new compound, glutathione is also a part of yet another potent antioxidant. This antioxidant has an extremely weird name; it is glutathione S-transferase. It's actually an enzyme, and what this antioxidant enzyme does aid in liver detoxification.

You may be thinking glutathione does a great job at protecting individual cells; however it also protects entire groups of cells at once. Aside from protecting a group of cells it also aids in protecting tissue in your brain, arteries, heart, immune cells, your lungs, liver, as well as kidneys and eye lenses. Talk about a variety of roles, and we're not finished yet!

It is widely thought that glutathione can prevent cancer. It is believed this antioxidant has the ability to scavenge carcinogens in your body! When it finds a cancer cell, glutathione transforms the carcinogen into a water-soluble object and helps your body in turn excrete the now water-soluble carcinogen!

A final property of glutathione makes a lot of sense and could show the most evidence into glutathione's antioxidant abilities. Many in the science and biology fields believe that glutathione can slow down and even potentially reverse the aging process. I'm not saying you'll lose years, however you may reduce the effects of aging. The reason this comes into belief is that as we age, the concentration of glutathione in our cells becomes more and more depleted. There's also a growing belief that this could potentially be a factor in why the elderly get sick faster. Talk about a correlation.

Green Tea

Green tea is probably one of the most popular antioxidants we know of and have studied. What book would this be without talking about green tea? Green tea is naturally full of plant based compounds called polyphenols. Polyphenols are phytonutrients (plant based nutrients). The most discussed polyphenol in green tea is epigallocatechin gallate. To save your eye site I'll refer to it as EGCG.

What makes EGCG so interesting is that it, similar to a select few amino acids, is able to seemingly sneak through cells. The main purpose in EGCG sneaking through bodily cells is that it can then form a sheath, or shield, DNA. When this polyphenol does this it aids in helping maintain DNA and prevent it from becoming damaged by hydrogen peroxide. When doing this, the DNA is not as easily damaged and may prevent the cellular mutation common in cancer growth.

Green tea polyphenols are also known to provide numerous heart healthy benefits such as potentially lowering cholesterol. Aside from this, another circulatory benefit provided by green tea is that it can reduce the amount blood clots.

Those with diabetes type 2 may see the greatest benefit from green tea. Green tea has shown in a multitude of studies to actually regulate insulin levels. In addition, diabetics may also notice that their blood sugar is held more in check and fluctuates much less. This is another trademark benefit of green tea.

Seeing many believe Type 2 diabetes is a lifestyle condition, it should be interesting to note that there is a reason many weight loss products promote their use of green tea. Instead of simply heating up your body (thermogenesis) green tea may actually melt areas of fat, helping them be utilized more efficiently as energy.

Melatonin

When I learned melatonin was could act as an antioxidant, I was shocked. Not because of the name or anything along those lines, but that it does not relate to what melatonin is known for one bit!

Melatonin is known to induce sleep. In fact, when I was drinking a ton of caffeine a day I used to pop 3 mgs of melatonin nightly so I could fall asleep. Reading into melatonin out of curiosity (to understand how it helped people sleep better) I found it was a potent antioxidant.

Think fast about extremists again (going back to our comparison between sickness/free radicals and how to fight them). If you look at the word as an amount, extremist is singular, right? Keep that in mind as the way melatonin works (as an antioxidant) may be a bit tricky. I'll tie it together for you at the end.

Melatonin is a pineal hormone, which means it is produced through the pineal gland. This hormone is very effective at scavenging and neutralizing free radicals. There's also something known as a singlet oxygen. Now we're going to look into something.

Oxygen is good, and oxygen molecules are very beneficial. Sometimes they can have negative side effects, which is where the singlet oxygen molecule comes in. This nasty little fellow is an "excited" oxygen molecule. Stay with me, I'll explain it. This "excited molecule" can cause damage to cellular membranes in turn potentially leading to cancer.

To make the idea of the singlet oxygen molecule more understandable, we're going to pose a scenario using radicals in the world of terror. You have a city, and in this city there is no known terror organization. There is one extremely radicalized individual who does not follow the cultural norms. He begins setting off explosions and causing problems. In your body that one radical individual is the singlet oxygen molecule, make sense now?

Another example could be a "wannabe" gang member in a rural town. Using the same idea, he robs and mugs people when they are walking. This is where melatonin is going to come in. Imagine in that town there is one police officer who knows gang activity inside and out. He notices this individual and without a doubt he goes after him and the "wannabe" gang member is now detained and can do no more harm.

Now that you understand why melatonin is important in defeating or "quenching" the harmful singlet oxygen molecules, let's look at another way melatonin can help you in other antioxidant ways. Let's look at the mitochondria again.

Very few things can permeate cells easily, getting through to the mitochondria can be a much more difficult task. You probably remember the mitochondria being the cells energy factory, or power plant for another way to look at it. Imagine an intruder breaking into a power plant and sabotaging a generator. Although the plant probably has 80 more, it obviously needs this generator.

Your body is the same with mitochondria, so if a free radical or "intruder" breaks into your internal energy supply it could cause havoc. In this case I want you to imagine melatonin being a highly trained security guard. This security guard will protect the generators before an intruder breaks in, right? Melatonin does the same thing to your mitochondria which is how it can pass through and protects them so effectively.

Many studies are done in non-human environments, either in a Petri dish or on mice (hence the term lab rat). Some studies regarding melatonin show extreme positive benefits, but keep in mind they are not in human clinical trials. Take a peek at them anyway as a lot of the mice studies over time have shown an ability to have very similar if not the same results in humans.

One of the studies done on mice has shown true antioxidant properties, at very effective rates. Melatonin has shown in lab studies on mice to prevent and inhibit cancer growth (think back to how melatonin fights singlet oxygen molecules). It also has shown the ability to protect against degenerative diseases and modulate the mice's immune systems.

N-Acetylcysteine

N-Acetylcysteine was one of my favorite supplements growing up and being involved in athletics. I began smoking at an early age and obviously ran into the problems with breathing, but I loved smoking. Someone told me about N-Acetylcysteine (we'll call in NAC) and that if I smoke I should take it. After a week on it, my lungs felt as if I had never smoked a day in my life!

NAC is a byproduct of an amino acid known as cysteine (if you look, you can see the relationship to the parent nutrient in NAC's name - sort of like having mommy's nose). Your body needs cysteine to be able to help it produce glutathione (which we mentioned earlier in this book) which is an extremely potent antioxidant and free radical killer. Because cysteine can be a very unstable amino acid and may not be the best thing to count on, NAC becomes even more beneficial as it is a much more stable compound.

Being the geek, I wanted to know why they recommend NAC and I began looking into it. NAC has a long history of being thought to help with respiratory issues like chronic bronchitis and COPD. I read that it could also be very beneficial to those with asthma.

What I wasn't told as it can benefit those around cigarette smoke is that NAC can be beneficial in reducing the harmful effects of secondhand smoke! NAC also acts as an extremely effective detoxifier.

Speaking of detoxifier, your lymphocytes and liver find NAC really helpful. They use it to prevent damage from all sorts of toxic compounds and poisons. This is where the benefit of fighting second hand smoke effects comes in. NAC is known to help detoxify alcohol, cigarette smoke, and other pollutants in the environment which are known to bring down the effectiveness of your immune system.

A last known benefit of NAC is that it slows down cellular damage, which we have seen in a few other antioxidants. This not only prevents cellular mutations but preserves their strength as well as fighting off aging. Along with that, chronic issues (similar to chronic bronchitis, but on a deeper level) have issues beating the helpful benefits of NAC as it reduces how often infectious diseases can inflict their wrath on you and shortens their lifespan.

Nicotinamide Adenine Dinucleotide (NADH)

NADH does not have the luxury of being one of the more studied antioxidants, and therefore has some of the least knowledge into its benefits. That's not to say you shouldn't consider it at all though! In fact this is what helps many cells come into being!

Going back to cancer, we know it can be spawned from damaged DNA. Let's go back to our war on terror example. After the troops have salvaged the remains of a city and protected the inhabitants form an attack, there is still a damaged infrastructure. This is where NADH is known to come in. It will help by repairing the damaged buildings (DNA) from the free radicals attacks.

Oligomeric Proanthocyanidins

Say that antioxidant 30 times fast, I bet you'll end up with a knot in your tongue. Truth be told you wouldn't want to tease this antioxidant about its name, oligomeric proanthocyanidins.

Imagine someone with a real geeky name where you just visualize them being a 90 pound, pimple faced, book nerd and that book nerd ends up actually being a JV All Pro defensive end that towers over 6'6 and 300 pounds. This funny name packs an incredible antioxidant "punch".

I'll also mention that if you haven't read my book on Flavonoids (you really should, it is INSERT FLAVONOID BOOK HERE), is that they contain a compound known as anthocyanidins. If you look at the name of this antioxidant closely, oligomeric proanthocyanidins, you will notice what they truly are. They are a form of the phytonutrient flavonoids. Being said, you're able to find them naturally in specific plants or living things.

Like flavonoids, you will also be able to obtain these through different forms and there are two extremely popular types. The first type is from pine bark extract; however the more popular form is from grape seed extract. If you pay attention to health at all, you will know that grape seed extract is known for numerous health benefits. Now you know why, and you will read more about them in the following write up on oligomeric proanthocyanidins.

Aside from simply saying this antioxidant is packing an extremely potent punch, let's go a bit further and compare it to vitamin C and even vitamin E. OPC (oligomeric proanthocyanidins using its initials) is thought to make the known and massive benefits of the mentioned vitamins appear miniscule. In fact, some studies are suggesting it can be 50 times more powerful than vitamin E and 20 times more potent than vitamin C.

In our everyday life, there are some things that are too good to be thrown out, right? Even with shampoo bottles we can add a little bit of water to get a few more uses out, and in turn save a few dollars. We reheat leftovers and can make them into another meal by using them properly as well. Remember those two examples as they can be seen as an analogy in how our body and glutathione can use vitamin C.

I'm going to cover the antioxidant power of vitamin C later on, but one thing I'd like to explain is that it is excreted when it is deemed "unusable" or no longer needed by our bodies.

Wouldn't it be cool if you could reuse your vitamin C? If you're thinking I am about to tell you how you can you are correct! Along with being more potent than vitamin C, OPC's can help with vitamin C being salvaged and reused in your body. OPCs have the ability to increase the already potent antioxidant effects of oxidized vitamin C by aiding glutathione in recycling the vitamin before it is excreted by your body.

Yet another benefit of the antioxidant OPC is how they are able to pass your brain's blood-brain barrier. With their ability to do this, OPCs can also aid in helping to protect both your brain as well as the nerves in your spine from the onslaught of free radical attacks. Think of this as a specialized force breaking past an enclosed or barricaded center of a town and fighting the intruders in there.

Something about OPCs that I found interesting was their effect on something I had been dealing with my whole life. Aside from aging more rapidly due to my cigarette smoking (they help slow the aging process as well), OPCs can hamper the effects you feel with allergies. They do this little trick by reducing histamine production in your body which is thought to be responsible for allergic as well as inflammatory responses, both of which are not very pleasant.

One allergy (type I should say) I have is to a number of foods, including some of which can cause a fatal allergic reaction (peanut oil, walnuts, etc.). I have not seen any compelling evidence toward which allergy OPCs are known to help diminish the effects of.

Selenium

To me, selenium was always a mineral. I'll give it credit it is an essential trace mineral, but for years I always just rang it up (while working with nutritional supplements) without giving it much thought. One day, I remember speaking with a customer about it and they asked me why in the antioxidant section it always had vitamin E with it. I looked into it and found I wasn't just ringing up an essential trace mineral, but rather a massive antioxidant!

When I looked into the customer's question, I realized why there was selenium in the mineral section and then selenium in the antioxidant section. Although selenium is a potent antioxidant, it does not work alone. In fact, to really see the powers selenium has to offer you need to have it in conjunction with vitamin E.

When selenium is partnered with vitamin E, you see some regular tasks being handled such as protecting cells as well as cell membranes from free radical damage. Something on top of that protective attribute is that selenium (with vitamin E) can also work to increase the antioxidant levels inside of individual cells.

I had mentioned earlier about the antioxidant glutathione peroxidase. Selenium is a key contributor to that enzyme coming into existence and being a potent antioxidant on its own.

Selenium, although essential, is not particularly difficult to incorporate into your diet. Plants like asparagus (I won't eat the stuff due to bad childhood memories, I still get the shivers), garlic, and a wide variety of grains (such as buckwheat and brown rice) contain good selenium levels. How much selenium you will get from these veggies and grains is obviously going to be dependent on how much selenium is is in the soil the plants use as a nutrient.

If you go and buy an over the counter selenium supplement, you may notice it is near impossible to find one with more than 400 micrograms per serving. There's a lot of sense into that, too much selenium can actually be toxic.

Many multivitamins (especially since developing countries are on an antioxidant kick) actually have selenium listed. One thing you should consider about multivitamins is that they are not a "one size fits all" type of supplement. In my experience and studies, you're certainly going to be getting what you pay for.

Silymarin

The name of this antioxidant may sound funny (much like OPC's real name), however I have seen this antioxidant do some serious damage (to bad things in a good way that is! Silymarin is an extract from an herb called milk thistle (silymarin actually comes from the seed of this herb) and is older than the USA in how long it's been used in medical practices.

Something special about silymarin is the fact this extract provides a ton of very powerful and extremely potent antioxidants. Because this is a plant based super food, I'm going to have to assume you know that the main nutrients are flavonoid based, and if you didn't know that now you do.

As mentioned, silymarin has been used medicinally by numerous cultures. Its main focal point is on the liver. The liver helps your body filter just about everything; this means it is very vulnerable to free radical attacks, "pollution", buildups, and everything else you can imagine. Silymarin aids your liver against those attacks. On top of that silymarin also helps your liver promote new cells.

Aside from being a chronic smoker, I was also an extremely heavy drinker; by extremely heavy I mean 2 bottles of gin a day. I started to show signs of aging and upon visiting a naturopath friend of mine received a bottle of milk thistle seed extract. I looked at him funny and he mentioned that a habitual drinker such as myself would benefit greatly from the extract.

After I quit drinking and began using the Milk Thistle Seed extract my routine blood work showed something very off. It appeared my liver was fully functional and had amazing levels of everything it helped produce. What they were, I do not remember. What I do remember is becoming a lifelong user of this herb with a very funny name.

Superoxide Dismutase

Based on what we know about free radicals, you may be thinking I made a mistake as this is clearly not an antioxidant. In fact, you are incorrect (but good job remember many free radicals have oxide in their name). In fact, superoxide dismutase is an extremely potent antioxidant! this enzyme actually does some extremely important things to your body. Maybe not to your body, but inside of it.

Firstly, superoxide dismutase (we'll call it SOD from here on) helps to revitalize your cells from free radical attacks while also slowing down the rate of attack from the (what many consider) most dangerous free radical in your body superoxide radical. Think of SOD and superoxide radicals as twins where one fights for good the other for death. In that situation, SOD fights for good and tries to protect and kill superoxide radical.

SOD is being looked into for its anti aging potential benefits. SOD also slowly begins to decrease as we age. This should come as no surprise since free radical "attacks" become more frequent and severe as we get older.

We need some minerals to be absorbed (not to be confused with heavy metals) so that we can function properly. SOD helps our bodies utilize these very important minerals effectively. With that being mentioned, SOD comes in two forms.

The first form of SOD I'll discuss is the one that works with copper and zinc. What this particular form does is add a sort of "fortification" of antioxidant protection into the watery part around cells, this is called cytoplasm. When stuff happens inside of the cytoplasm, you get free radical creation. When the free radicals are being created, SOD quickly takes them out before they can cause harm in your body.

The other form of SOD deals with manganese. Like the copper/zinc form this is also active in cells, however its area of focus lays in your mitochondria. If you remember, this is where energy is produced. This is obviously going to lead to the creation of free radicals, and again this form of SOD comes in quickly and kills off the potential cell attackers.

You may be wondering where you can get SOD from, because like all humans you have cytoplasm as well as mitochondria you'd like protected. A lot of green plants carry this enzyme such as broccoli, sprouts, cabbage, wheatgrass, and many more.

Vitamin A (Plus Carotenoids)

I've combined these two because in essence, they work together. With that being said, the way they work together is many carotenoids (roughly 50, which is 10% of the known carotenoids) convert into vitamin A inside your body.

Carotenoids are a phytonutrient that have some extreme antioxidant powers. Since I mentioned they are phytonutrients, we know they're from plants. If it makes sense, they actually are pigments inside of red, orange, yellow and some green plants. They're mainly the bright and flamboyant colored plants.

Another thing about carotenoid phytonutrients is they are fat soluble, just like vitamin A! The main carotenoids that have been studied are alpha and beta (two different carotenoids) carotene, lutein, lycopene, as well as zeaxanthin.

I've touched on singlet oxygen molecules and stated they are similar to, but are not free radicals. They are however extremely reactive and can damage other molecules. Carotenoids come in and quench these bad boys before they can begin to do serious damage to other body cells.

I've done some extensive research into carotenoids, because as a smoker some of them could actually cause me more harm than good! For instance, carotenoids have some extremely potent anticancer properties. For smokers though, they can actually increase my risk of conditions such as lung cancer.

I mentioned I was afraid of getting cancer due to supplementation with carotenoids. If you're not a smoker, carotenoids could be extremely beneficial to your health! It is thought that alpha and beta carotene, lycopene, as well as lutein have the ability to reduce the oxidative damage inflicted by free radicals and singlet oxygen molecules. What this does is protect your DNA.

Have you ever heard that vitamin A is good for your eyes? Another effect of carotenoids (don't forget, many can be converted into vitamin A in our body through a metabolic process) is that it helps fight against among other things age related macular degeneration as well as cataracts.

If you want to hear a wholesome story of teamwork, ALA, CoQ10, and vitamins C and E can work together to keep carotenoids inside of your body tissues. If this doesn't speak to the importance of carotenoids I don't know what does!

I mentioned some carotenoids can be converted by your body into vitamin A. One such carotenoid is alpha-carotene. When your body doesn't need any more alpha-carotene to be converted to vitamin A, you will begin to use it as an antioxidant. What this new antioxidant does is prevent cholesterol in your body from becoming oxidized as well as breaking up free radical chain reactions.

I mentioned there are a wide range of plants that contain high levels of carotenoids, and it'd be a pain for you to read every single one of them. What I'll do is I'll tell you which plants contain the highest levels of carotenoids, fair enough (I read feedback, literally just let me know you want a full list and you have it!)? Some great sources of carotenoids in plants are spirulina, corn, sweet peppers (all colors), spinach, kale, and sweet potatoes. If I were you I'd start adding them to your diet!

Before I move on, let me tell you why you may want to have them dietarily. A big reason is that too much carotenoids in one serving can actually have adverse reactions in your body. There was a study that stated if you're taking in more than 50,000 I.U.'s (International Units) of beta-carotene you could start screwing around with your natural cell division.

Vitamin C

Unless you've been living under a nutritional rock (if they existed), you know that vitamin C helps your immune system dramatically. We've also learned that vitamin C is not the most powerful antioxidant there is, which even surprised myself and I've read into health topics quite a bit. Regardless, vitamin C is needed by your body for a variety of functions, and not all of them are due to its antioxidant properties!

Skipping ahead of vitamin C's antioxidant potency, I'll cover some other things vitamin C does for your body. Vitamin C helps you prevent against nasty stuff such as atherosclerosis by protecting your cell walls from being damaged! Let' get into why it's important as an antioxidant, especially since this is an antioxidant book.

Let's first look at our body as a fortress (because I'm a geek and I think the fighting analogies are awesome). We have walls of defense and we have main areas we cannot afford to have damaged. Our control tower is going to be our brain and spinal column.

Our brain and spinal column are under constant attack by free radicals, you can say they are constantly waging attacks on them and be correct. High amounts of vitamin C can protect your control center (like a lot of milligrams high amounts).

Vitamin C is also a water soluble vitamin. What this means is due to vitamin C's water soluble nature it is able to go into body fluids and start attack free radicals before they can cause serious damage. Imagining your body as a fortress again, vitamin C is your fortress' first line of defense!

One thing I have learned about vitamin C, actually 2 things, are that something can help it become absorbed better and something can help it fight off free radicals better. Hesperidin is a phytonutrient and helps vitamin C fight off free radicals more effectively. Also, when it comes to absorbing vitamin C it may be beneficial to take it with rose hips or other bioflavonoids.

Vitamin E

Vitamin E is a fat soluble vitamin, and it is also a very potent antioxidant. We know that oxidation of things in our body can cause severe issues overtime. Vitamin E helps to fight the oxidation of fats.

Atherosclerosis is a bad thing; it's when fat has been oxidized (overtime, not at once). We need fats though; our cell membranes are composed of them! Free radical attack can make that fat go rancid. This is a big benefit of vitamin E being fat soluble comes in. What this does is it allows vitamin E to protect the cells coating from, in essence, going bad.

Something really neat I found out about vitamin E is that on top of helping protect your cell membranes and their coating it also helps with using oxygen. As I mentioned vitamin E could be tied in with helping your body fight off atherosclerosis, it should make sense to know that vitamin E is also effective against coronary artery disease.

Let's look at 2 little know facts about vitamin E. The first fact is that zinc could be needed to maintain optimal vitamin E levels in your body. Speaking of maintaining vitamin E in your body, you may also need selenium to enhance it properties. This makes sense due to the fact in your body, selenium and vitamin E work together. One other very interesting fact about vitamin E is the forms it comes in. When reading a nutritional label, you will notice something when looking at vitamin E. Often times it seems as if companies accidentally place an l next to the d. You may see d-alpha-tocopherol and you may also see dl-alpha-tocopherol. There is no mistake actually and they are both vitamin E, but one is better than the other. D-alpha-tocopherol (missing the l) is the natural form and is thought to be far superior to the synthetic or manmade form.

Vitamin E can be added to your diet aside from supplementation. You can in fact get vitamin E through soybeans (which have a TON of other amazing nutrients), sunflower seeds, sweet potatoes, as well as asparagus.

So Which Antioxidant Should You Take?

You're going to have to agree with me that the question leading off this ending and short chapter is going to be nearly impossible to answer. Which one do you want to talk to your doctor most about? That is still nearly impossible to answer. I'm not a doctor however I realize certain activities, environments, even lines of work can pose risks to us on a variety of levels.

Your doctor isn't going to tell you not to take an antioxidant (and if you're not suffering a serious condition, I'd really seek a second opinion). But letting them know about you and your life is instrumental in finding a good combination of antioxidants. Combination, you may be wondering? Let's take a peek at why a combination of smaller doses may be beneficial.

Antioxidants perform different roles and do different things. You know this as you've just read this short read! I've listed the antioxidants in this book that I have witnessed and heard testimony to working the best. Carotenoids do different things than flavonoids, right? Why take one over the other? A garlic supplement (unless AGE) may not be needed as your doctor could tell you to stop being so lazy and cook using more garlic.

There are numerous awesome antioxidant combinations from a company I Personally love called Daniel Chapter One. I have seen firsthand the effect their products can have on individuals as compared to "leading brands". The founder knows how things work on a bimolecular level, and due to their products I feel my asthma as well as my allergies have become a thing of the past. Do I still cough and sneeze? Of course, I smoke cigarettes. However I do know I am not getting an allergy shot once a month, even sometimes twice a week! Personally I attribute it to that company.

I still use multiple products from Daniel Chapter One, and although I get nothing for mentioning them, I can tell you I would recommend as someone who has used them you do the same. Look up Daniel Chapter One in Portsmouth, Rhode Island.

Important, Not Reading This Could Kill You!

I am not a doctor, I will not portray myself to be one nor will I attempt to consider diagnosing your long-term aches or sniffles. I have no medical training and cannot be held liable for you making unwise decisions based on what you read. This book should be considered as educational purposes only!

Your primary doctor knows your situation and knows you better than most do. Stopping a treatment program could possibly kill you. Going against their orders could possibly kill you. Getting a second opinion, however, will not kill you. You must get that second opinion from someone who is licensed medically.

Let me break it down further, just in case. I DO NOT KNOW YOU, unless you come to a book signing, I will not meet you. I cannot prescribe, diagnose, or cure anything with you or in general (although I self diagnose regularly, it is mainly stress stemmed from the fact I have a child's mother who is "not all there", again I know my situation not yours). Your doctor is not against you helping yourself, in fact with certain cholesterol lowering drugs they may actually RECOMMEND you take an antioxidant listed!

Just because an antioxidant is listed and the properties and ways to help you seem great, you could be harmed if they interact adversely with your medicine. This is not good and could kill you.

Think first, ask your doctor second, act third. Doing anything in that order that relates directly to your health will save you insane amounts of pain and suffering in the future!

Why Listen to Me (A Short Autobiography to offer me some "Cred") If I'm Not Practicing Medicine?

I remember the first time I had heard the term antioxidant, and I remember how I laughed at it. It was shortly after my kindergarten graduation ceremony. It was a private ceremony. The only people there were my teacher, my principal, my mom and grandmother. Father Folster was there too and he promised me a ride in a fire truck, when I got better.

The reason I had a priest there wasn't because just because I was graduating from a Catholic school. The reason I was having a private graduation wasn't because I am something special (although we all are). I loved fire trucks. I had actually graduated kindergarten, that's why my former principal and teacher were there. My grandmother and mom were there because they never left me. I was dying. Father Folster was there as it was common, he was also there giving me the sacrament of the Last Rites. I was going to leave the ICU and become a soldier, albeit a very young soldier, in my God's army.

I didn't die, obviously because I am now writing this in my 30's and I do not believe in reincarnation, because I couldn't. I remember the nurse telling me why I had to eat the fruit I didn't want to eat. It had antioxidants and they were going to help me get better, when I got better my Grammy and mom wouldn't have to worry and cry when I was sleeping at night anymore. Antioxidants were going to heal me!

Truth be told, I think a lot of it had to do with the medicine they kept giving me along with the care of the nurses, doctors, and especially my family. But I was sold on the idea antioxidants were something I needed to eat.

Through the years, I knew how to become "anti sick". I also knew how to take poison ivy and rub it all over my face to miss school so I could read more (except one time when my eyes wouldn't open -oops). That carried into my 2 favorite jobs, an assistant manager and very high selling associate at a nutritional chain and a fitness center tri owner (with a two other family members).

What I saw day in and day out in those two jobs was remarkable. I saw what the power of antioxidants could do to people. Survival stories led me to have a conviction and determination to know all I could about health, and spread that knowledge.

I never attained a medical degree because honestly, school wasn't for me. I wanted my own curriculum, plus having children at a young age and years of trouble making kind of halted my chances. I guess I could now, but I honestly find immense joy instead in giving you what I think and know. With that being said, I am not a doctor at any kind. This book is for informational purposes only (even though I said that, we need to make sure we communicate with our doctor before doing things).

www.ingramcontent.com/pod-product-compliance
Lightning Source LLC
Chambersburg PA
CBHW070334290526
45791CB00003B/1329